FIBROIDS

HOW TO PROPERLY DEAL WITH FIBROIDS

DR. PAT DANIEL

Contents

CHAPTER ONE

INTRODUCTION

Fibroids in the uterus are tumors that expand in or at the walls of the uterus. They may be common and no longer typically cancerous. Fibroids do now not continuously cause symptoms, but can motive pain and bleeding.

Fibroids inside the uterus, or uterine fibroids, are the most commonplace noncancerous, or benign, tumors in people of childbearing age. They may be moreover called leiomyomas and myomas.

Many people have fibroids and now not using a symptoms and signs, while others experience pain, bleeding, or each.

Uterine fibroids are a commonplace form of noncancerous tumor that would broaden in and in your uterus. Not all fibroids reason signs, however after they do, symptoms can encompass heavy menstrual bleeding, once more pain, frequent urination and pain all through intercourse. Small fibroids often don't need treatment, but large fibroids can be dealt with with medicinal drugs or surgical remedy.

Uterine fibroids (additionally referred to as leiomyomas) are growths fabricated from muscle and tissue that form in or at the wall of your uterus. Those growths are generally now not cancerous (benign) and are the most not unusual noncancerous tumor in women and people assigned girl at transport (AFAB).

Uterine fibroids can purpose a spread of signs and symptoms like ache and heavy, irregular vaginal bleeding. Occasionally, a person has no symptoms and is unaware they have got fibroids. Treatment for fibroids generally depends for your signs and symptoms and signs.

Uterine fibroids are noncancerous growths of the uterus that frequently seem throughout childbearing years. Additionally referred to as leiomyomas (lie-o-my-O-muhs) or myomas, uterine fibroids are not associated with an elevated threat of uterine maximum cancers and nearly in no way grow to be maximum cancers.

Fibroids range in size from seedlings, undetectable by means of using the human eye, to cumbersome hundreds that could distort and increase the uterus. You could have a single fibroid or a couple of ones. In severe cases, more than one fibroids can increase the uterus plenty that it reaches the rib cage and can add weight.

Many women have uterine fibroids someday at some stage in their lives. However you may not apprehend you have were given uterine fibroids due to the fact they often cause no signs and symptoms. Your health practitioner might also discover fibroids incidentally at some stage in a pelvic examination or prenatal ultrasound.

Uterine fibroids, which your medical doctor

can also call leiomyomas or myomas, are tumors manufactured from muscle that may grow in your uterus. They rarely emerge as cancer. And in case you get them, it doesn't imply you're more likely to get uterine maximum cancers.

Fibroids can range plenty in duration, shape, and location. They may display up to your uterus, uterine wall, or on its floor. They can also hook up with your uterus thru a stalk- or stem-like structure.

A few are so small that your medical doctor can't even see them with the naked eye. Others develop in large masses that may have an impact on the scale and form of your uterus.

Uterine fibroids normally appear even as

you're of childbearing age -- commonly among 30-40 years antique -- but they might show up at any age. They're more commonplace in Black humans than in white people. In addition they typically generally tend to show up earlier and increase faster in Black human beings. Docs don't understand why.

Wherein do fibroids increase?

Fibroids can expand as a unmarried nodule (one boom) or in a cluster. Clusters of fibroids can range in length from 1 millimeter to more than 20 centimeters (eight inches) in diameter or maybe big. For evaluation, fibroids may be as small as a seed or get as massive as a watermelon. The ones growths can increase inside the wall of your uterus, inside the primary hollow space of your uterus or at the outer ground of your uterus.

Sorts of uterine fibroids

There are fantastic forms of uterine fibroids counting on wherein they're placed and how they join. Specific forms of uterine fibroids include:

Intramural fibroids: the ones fibroids are embedded into the muscular wall of your uterus. They're the most not unusual type.

Submucosal fibroids: those fibroids grow below the internal lining of your uterus.

Subserosal fibroids: This form of fibroid grows beneath the lining of the outer floor of your uterus. They may end up quite huge and turn into your pelvis.

Pedunculated fibroids: The least not unusual type, those fibroids connect in your uterus with a stalk or stem. They're frequently defined as mushroom-like because they've a stalk after which a far broader pinnacle.

Are fibroids not unusual?

Fibroids are a totally commonplace sort of increase. Approximately 40% to 80% of humans with a uterus have fibroids. They stand up most usually in people among 30 and 50 years antique. Those who haven't had their first duration (menstruation) however commonly don't have fibroids. They're additionally less common in people who've entered menopause.

Many ladies who've fibroids haven't any symptoms. In folks who do, signs may be inspired via the area, duration and type of fibroids.

In women who have symptoms, the most common signs and symptoms and signs and symptoms and signs and symptoms of uterine fibroids consist of:

Heavy menstrual bleeding

Menstrual periods lasting more than every week

Pelvic pressure or pain

Common urination

Trouble emptying the bladder

Constipation

Backache or leg pains

Hardly ever, a fibroid can purpose acute ache at the same time as it outgrows its blood deliver, and starts offevolved to die.

Fibroids are usually labeled with the useful resource of their place. Intramural fibroids grow within the muscular uterine wall. Submucosal fibroids bulge into the uterine cavity. Subserosal fibroids assignment to the outside of the uterus.

Motives of Uterine Fibroids

Specialists don't recognize precisely why you get fibroids. Hormones and genetics might make you more likely to get them.

CHAPTER TWO

Hormones. Estrogen and progesterone are the hormones that make the lining of your uterus thicken each month at some point of your duration. Additionally they appear to have an effect on fibroid boom. At the same time as hormone manufacturing slows down at some point of menopause, fibroids typically shrink.

Genetics. Researchers have positioned genetic variations among fibroids and everyday cells inside the uterus.

Different boom factors. Substances on your frame that assist with tissue protection, such as insulin-like boom element, may additionally moreover play a factor in fibroid increase.

Extracellular matrix (ECM). ECM makes your cells stick collectively. Fibroids have extra ECM than normal cells, which makes them fibrous or ropey. ECM additionally shops increase elements (substances that spur mobile boom) and reasons cells to change.

What does uterine fibroid pain feel like?

There are a selection of feelings you would likely enjoy when you have fibroids. When you have small fibroids, you could experience nothing in any respect and no longer even phrase they're there. For large fibroids, however, you may experience pain and ache. Fibroids can purpose you to experience again ache, stabbing pains for your belly or even ache throughout intercourse.

What do fibroids seem like?

Fibroids are commonly rounded growths that appear to be smooth bumps. In some cases, they'll be connected with a thin stem, giving them a mushroom-like appearance.

At the same time as to peer a scientific physician

See your physician when you have:

Pelvic pain that doesn't depart

Overly heavy, prolonged or painful periods

Recognizing or bleeding among durations

Difficulty emptying your bladder

Unexplained low purple blood cellular depend (anemia)

Are attempting to find set off health facility remedy if you have intense vaginal bleeding or sharp pelvic ache that comes on.

Hazard factors of Uterine Fibroids

A few things can boom your possibilities of having uterine fibroids, collectively with:

Age

Race

Getting your duration at a younger age

Delivery manage use

Diet D deficiency

Ingesting an excessive amount of pork and

not enough inexperienced veggies, fruit, or dairy

Alcohol

Own family records

You're more likely to get fibroids if close loved ones like your mother or sister have had them.

What are the complications of uterine fibroids?

Maximum uterine fibroids don't cause severe headaches. However, the most not unusual headaches of fibroids are:

Pain that becomes unmanageable.

Swelling of your stomach or pelvic vicinity.

Immoderate bleeding.

Anemia.

Infertility (this is uncommon).

Can fibroids cause anemia?

Anemia is a condition that takes place at the same time as your frame doesn't have sufficient healthy crimson blood cells to maintain oxygen in your organs. Anemia can display as much as human beings who've frequent or distinctly heavy durations. Fibroids can reason your intervals to be very heavy or so that you can even bleed among periods. Talk to your healthcare issuer in case you're experiencing signs and symptoms of anemia at the same time as you have fibroids.

Uterine Fibroid prognosis

Your doctor may additionally suspect you've got were given uterine fibroids really from feeling your uterus sooner or later of a ordinary pelvic exam. If the form of your uterus feels irregular or notably huge, they'll order further checks, together with:

Ultrasound. Ultrasounds use sound waves to take a photo of your uterus. A technician will place a tool both on your vagina or for your stomach to get the pictures. Then your clinical doctor can see if you have fibroids and wherein and the way huge they're.

Lab checks. Your medical doctor might also want you to have blood exams to help decide out why you've got fibroids. Your whole blood depend (CBC) can assist them determine whether you have anemia (low tiers of crimson blood cells) or special bleeding problems.

Magnetic resonance imaging (MRI). If your health practitioner wishes more statistics after you've got an ultrasound, you could additionally have an MRI. MRIs show extra certain pics of fibroids and may assist medical doctors determine the exquisite remedy. Your medical health practitioner can also recommend an MRI when you have a big uterus or are close to menopause.

Hysterosonography. In this test, a technician pushes a small amount of saline answer into your uterine hole space to make it large. This helps them see fibroids which might be growing into your uterus (submucosal fibroids) and the liner of your uterus. This is useful in case you're seeking to get pregnant or have heavy durations.

Hysterosalpingography. In case your medical doctor desires to look if your fallopian tubes are blocked, you might have a hysterosalpingography. Your physician uses dye to focus on your uterus and fallopian tubes on an X-ray to look these regions higher.

Hysteroscopy. Your scientific physician inserts a small telescope with a mild attached into your cervix. Then, after injecting saline and increasing your uterine cavity, they might have a have a look at the partitions of your uterus and fallopian tube beginning.

How are uterine fibroids dealt with?

Treatment for uterine fibroids can range relying on the scale, quantity and vicinity of the fibroids, in addition to what symptoms they're causing. If you aren't experiencing any symptoms from your fibroids, you cannot need treatment. Small fibroids can frequently be left by myself. A few humans by no means revel in any symptoms or have any troubles related to fibroids. In those cases, your employer can also advocate monitoring your fibroids with pelvic assessments or ultrasounds.

If you're experiencing symptoms from your

fibroids — which includes anemia from extra bleeding, slight to extreme pain or urinary tract and bowel troubles — you'll want remedy to assist. Your remedy plan will rely upon some factors, which incorporates:

How many fibroids you've got got.

The scale of your fibroids.

Wherein your fibroids are placed.

What signs you're experiencing associated with the fibroids.

Your choice to maintain your uterus.

The first-rate remedy desire for you may moreover rely on your plans for pregnancy within the future. Communicate in your healthcare issuer approximately your fertility dreams while discussing treatment alternatives. Treatment alternatives for uterine fibroids can include:

Medicinal pills

Over the counter (OTC) pain medicines: those medicines help manage pain and pain as a result of fibroids. OTC medicinal drugs embody acetaminophen and ibuprofen.

Iron nutritional dietary supplements: when you have anemia from extra bleeding, your provider can also propose you are taking an iron complement.

Start control: starting manipulate can also help with signs and symptoms of fibroids — especially, heavy bleeding at some point of and among intervals and menstrual cramps.

There are a spread of start manage alternatives you can use, which includes oral contraceptive drugs, jewelry, injections and intrauterine gadgets (IUDs).

Gonadotropin-liberating hormone (GnRH) agonists: those drug treatments paintings with the aid of shrinking fibroids. They're from time to time used to lessen a fibroid earlier than surgical procedure, making it less complicated to take away the fibroid. However, these medications are short, and if you prevent taking them, the fibroids can grow returned.

Oral treatment plans: Elagolix is a new oral remedy to manipulate heavy uterine bleeding in individuals who haven't experienced menopause with symptomatic uterine fibroids. It can be taken for as lots as 24 months. Communicate for your company approximately the professionals and cons of this remedy. Every other oral remedy, tranexamic acid, treats heavy menstrual bleeding in human beings with uterine fibroids.

It's important to talk in your healthcare organisation about any remedy you take. Constantly seek advice from your organisation earlier than beginning a brand new medicine to speak about any possible complications.

Fibroid surgical procedure

There are numerous factors to remember whilst speakme about the different sorts of surgical remedy for fibroid removal. Now not most effective can the size, vicinity and extensive form of fibroids have an impact at the form of surgical treatment, however your dreams for future pregnancies can also be an vital element at the same time as developing a remedy plan. Some surgical options hold your uterus and will let you turn out to be pregnant within the future, at the same time as other options can either harm or cast off your uterus.

Myomectomy is a way that permits your provider to dispose of the fibroids. There are various sorts of myomectomy. The sort of method that may fit top notch for you may depend on where your fibroids are located, how massive they're and how many you have. The varieties of myomectomy procedures to remove fibroids can encompass:

Hysteroscopy: Your employer inserts a scope (a skinny, bendy, tube-like tool) through your vagina and cervix and into your uterus. Your corporation uses the scope to cut away and get rid of the fibroids.

Laparoscopy: on this system, your corporation will use a scope to get rid of the fibroids. In assessment to hysteroscopy, this approach includes placing a few small incisions for your abdomen. That is how the scope will enter and go out your frame.

Laparotomy: at some stage in this process, your provider makes one huge incision on your belly and eliminates the fibroids thru this one lessen.

If you aren't planning future pregnancies, there are extra alternatives your healthcare issuer may also endorse. Those alternatives may be very effective, but they usually save you future pregnancies. Those can include:

Hysterectomy: Your employer gets rid of your uterus in the course of a hysterectomy. A hysterectomy is the fine manner to therapy fibroids. With the aid of getting rid of your uterus absolutely, the fibroids can't come decrease back and your signs and symptoms should go away. If your ovaries are left in region, you won't pass into menopause after a hysterectomy. This method might be endorsed in case you're experiencing very heavy bleeding out of your fibroids or if you have big fibroids. Minimally invasive hysterectomies encompass vaginal, laparoscopic or robotic techniques.

Uterine fibroid embolization: An interventional radiologist plays this manner with the assist of your gynecologist. They placed a small catheter on your uterine artery or radial artery and inject small debris, which then block the go with the flow of blood from the artery to the fibroids. Lack of blood drift shrinks the fibroids and improves your signs and signs. This technique may not be proper for all people.

Radiofrequency ablation (RFA): this is a secure and effective remedy that makes use of microwave (RF) strength to treat uterine fibroids. It's recommended for individuals who haven't reached menopause. It treats smaller fibroids.

CHAPTER THREE

Dangers to uterine fibroid remedy

There may be dangers to any remedy. Medicinal drugs may have facet outcomes and a few won't be an wonderful healthy for you. Speak to your healthcare issuer about all drug treatments you may be taking for other scientific conditions and your entire scientific history before beginning a new medicine. If you enjoy aspect effects after beginning a present day medicine, call your organization to talk about your alternatives.

There are also risks worried in surgical remedy of fibroids. Any surgical operation locations you liable to contamination and bleeding, and includes risks related to anesthesia. A in addition risk of fibroid removal surgical remedy can contain future pregnancies. Some surgical options can save you future pregnancies. Myomectomy is a manner that quality receives rid of the fibroids, taking into account destiny pregnancies. However, those who've had a myomectomy may additionally need to deliver destiny babies thru C-phase.

How huge do uterine fibroids want to be before being surgically removed?

There isn't a definitive length of a fibroid that might automatically propose it needs to be eliminated. Your healthcare agency will decide if surgical treatment is essential primarily based in your symptoms and symptoms. As an example, fibroids the dimensions of a small marble also can nonetheless cause excessive bleeding depending on their place. Your healthcare provider can talk signs and symptoms that would require surgical intervention.

What happens if fibroids pass untreated?

In case you don't have signs and symptoms, treatment for fibroids won't be important. If you have big fibroids or your signs are causing you ache and pain, getting treatment can be the tremendous choice. Most effective you and your issuer can determine the great route of treatment or if remedy is critical.

Prevention

No matter the truth that researchers preserve to examine the reasons of fibroid tumors, little clinical evidence is available on the way to prevent them. Stopping uterine fibroids may not be feasible, but best a small percentage of those tumors require remedy.

However, via making wholesome way of life selections, which include retaining a wholesome weight and eating fruits and veggies, you may be capable of lower your fibroid threat.

Additionally, a few studies suggests that the usage of hormonal contraceptives can be associated with a decrease danger of fibroids.

Can i get pregnant if i have uterine fibroids?

Sure, you may get pregnant if you have uterine fibroids. If you already apprehend you have got fibroids while you get pregnant, your healthcare provider will work with you to develop a monitoring plan for the fibroids. All through pregnancy, your body releases improved degrees of hormones. These hormones manual the pregnancy. However, they can also motive your fibroids to get larger. Huge fibroids can purpose the following issues sooner or later of pregnancy:

Elevated chance for a C-segment delivery due to the truth the fetus can't turn proper into a head-down role.

Hard work doesn't development.

Placental abruption.

Preterm delivery.

Can fibroids trade over the years?

Fibroids can without a doubt decrease or broaden through the years. They may trade length or frequently over an extended time period. This will appear for a spread of reasons, but in most times, this alteration in fibroid size is linked to the amount of hormones in your frame. When you have excessive tiers of hormones in your frame, fibroids can get large. This will arise at unique times to your existence, like throughout pregnancy. Fibroids can also reduce whilst your hormone ranges drop.

This is commonplace after menopause. Regularly, your signs and symptoms can also get better after menopause.

Will fibroids go away on their very very own?

Fibroids can reduce in a few people after menopause. This takes vicinity due to a decrease in hormones. When the fibroids lower, your signs and symptoms may match away. Small fibroids may not need treatment in the event that they aren't inflicting any signs and symptoms.

Do fibroids make you tired?

Feeling worn-out isn't a not unusual symptom of uterine fibroids. But, it's a commonplace symptom of anemia, that could arise while you lose an excessive amount of blood. Speak to a healthcare provider in case you experience excessively worn-out which will determine the purpose.

Do fibroids make your stomach massive?

Certain, it's viable that huge uterine fibroids can cause your stomach to bloat or seem big.

Conclusion

Uterine fibroids are a common scenario that many people enjoy in some unspecified time in the future in their lives. In a few cases, fibroids are small and don't purpose any signs and signs and symptoms in any respect. Different instances, fibroids can motive hard symptoms like pain and heavy vaginal bleeding. Speak to your healthcare company in case you revel in any sort of ache or ache. Fibroids are treatable.

THE END